Massimo Bolognesi

Silent myocardial ischemia in veteran athletes

AF153143

Massimo Bolognesi

Silent myocardial ischemia in veteran athletes

LAP LAMBERT Academic Publishing

Impressum / Imprint

Bibliografische Information der Deutschen Nationalbibliothek: Die Deutsche Nationalbibliothek verzeichnet diese Publikation in der Deutschen Nationalbibliografie; detaillierte bibliografische Daten sind im Internet über http://dnb.d-nb.de abrufbar.
Alle in diesem Buch genannten Marken und Produktnamen unterliegen warenzeichen-, marken- oder patentrechtlichem Schutz bzw. sind Warenzeichen oder eingetragene Warenzeichen der jeweiligen Inhaber. Die Wiedergabe von Marken, Produktnamen, Gebrauchsnamen, Handelsnamen, Warenbezeichnungen u.s.w. in diesem Werk berechtigt auch ohne besondere Kennzeichnung nicht zu der Annahme, dass solche Namen im Sinne der Warenzeichen- und Markenschutzgesetzgebung als frei zu betrachten wären und daher von jedermann benutzt werden dürften.

Bibliographic information published by the Deutsche Nationalbibliothek: The Deutsche Nationalbibliothek lists this publication in the Deutsche Nationalbibliografie; detailed bibliographic data are available in the Internet at http://dnb.d-nb.de.
Any brand names and product names mentioned in this book are subject to trademark, brand or patent protection and are trademarks or registered trademarks of their respective holders. The use of brand names, product names, common names, trade names, product descriptions etc. even without a particular marking in this work is in no way to be construed to mean that such names may be regarded as unrestricted in respect of trademark and brand protection legislation and could thus be used by anyone.

Coverbild / Cover image: www.ingimage.com

Verlag / Publisher:
LAP LAMBERT Academic Publishing
ist ein Imprint der / is a trademark of
OmniScriptum GmbH & Co. KG
Heinrich-Böcking-Str. 6-8, 66121 Saarbrücken, Deutschland / Germany
Email: info@lap-publishing.com

Herstellung: siehe letzte Seite /
Printed at: see last page
ISBN: 978-3-659-67480-8

Zugl. / Approved by: L'Aquila, University of L'Aquila, Diss., 2007

ACKNOWLEDGMENTS

My deepest gratitude to the many individuals who have made this Book-thesis

possible. First and foremost, recognition goes to the support staff of our institution for

their assistance with manuscript preparation and providing effective communication.

Heartfelt thanks to the many athletes who authorized us to publish their personal

data. Gratitude is well due to Olga Rusu, and the entire editorial and production

teams at LAP LAMBERT Academic Publishing for their professionalism and advice.

Finally, my sincere thanks go to my colleagues in General Practice Medicine and

Cardiology and above all to my family for their constant support and encouragement.

Contents

Introduction: the size of the problem (Pages 5 -9)

Investigation methods and accurate screening tests for Ischemic Coronary Disease (Pages 10 – 15)

1st Level Sport Medicine Assessment of a Master Athlete (35 years or over in age) professional competitor (Pages 16 – 20)

Personal Cases: experiences and management of silent ischemia cardiopathy of a primary level Sport Medicine Centre Survey (Pages 21 – 41)

True Positive (Pages 26 – 37)

False Positives (Pages 38-41)

Discussion (Pages 42 – 46)

Conclusion (Pages 47 - 49)

Bibliography (Pages 50 – 57)

GLOSSARY

AAFP: *American Academy of Family Physicians*

ACC/AHA: *American College of Cardiology/ American Heart Association*

ACP: *American College of Physicians*

BMI: *Body Mass Index*

CABG: *Coronary Artery Bypass Grafting*

COPD: *Chronic Obstructive Pulmonary Disease*

CHD: *Coronary Artery Disease*

CX: *Circumflex Coronary Artery*

CT: *Computerized Tomography*

DA: *Descending Artery*

ECG: *Electrocardiogram*

EF: *Ejection Fraction*

HDL: *High-density Lipoprotein*

HR: *Heart Rate*

LIMA: *Left Internal Mammary Artery*

ABP: *Arterial Blood Pressure*

METS: *Metabolic Equivalents*

MO: *Marginal Obtuse branch*

PTCA: *Percutaneous Transluminal Coronary Angioplasty*

PVCs: *Premature Ventricular Contractions*

SD: *Standard Deviation*

WHF: *World Health Federation*

VR: *Ventricular Repolarization*

Introduction: the size of the problem

The advances made in the last 30 years have dramatically changed the attitude of the medical community towards the relationship between physical activity and ageing. Regular physical activity is a prerequisite for a healthy life and postpones age-related disability. In aged people, it improves muscular strength, articular flexibility, balance, and promotes greater calcium fixation, consequently reducing the risk of bone fractures. More importantly, regular physical exercise contributes to the primary and secondary prevention of cardiovascular disease, diabetes, and dyslipidemias that are closely interrelated and negatively affected by sedentary lifestyle.

Sports physicians and cardiologists should have an unconditionally supportive attitude towards "competitive sports activity" programs. In middle-aged or elderly individuals, competitive sport is an irreplaceable stimulus to continue or pursue a lifestyle that promotes health and particularly, physical fitness. This is exemplified in the Master sports participants, an ever-growing category of athletes which accounts for 50% of sports federation membership in Italy. Master athletes are typically 35-40 years or older, and are engaged in competitive events organized by the sports federations affiliated to the Italian Olympic Committee (CONI). Masters compete in 5-year age group in many sports (triathlon, rowing, skiing, tennis, etc.), but most frequently in athletics (track & field events) (long distance running), cycling and swimming. In an evergrowing number of Master athletes, trainability does not differ from that of younger high-level athletes, pointing to an outstanding physiological model for the understanding of the aging process. For example, Master marathon runners at the top of world and national rankings show a 30-50% increase in VO^2 max compared to age-matched sedentary subjects. Despite a high, or sometimes outstanding, performance, the determination of eligibility to competitive sports is a delicate issue in these athletes. There is a fundamental difference between regular moderate, intensity in physical activity and competitive sports, in that the documented benefits of low-to-moderate intensity exercise is not associated with any additional risks, whereas competitive performance may create maximal

5

physical and psychological burden with increased risk of cardiovascular complications, including exercise-induced sudden cardiac death. The higher prevalence of coronary heart disease (CHD) with aging, even among asymptomatic patients, accounts for this phenomenon. The most prevalent complication of sports activity is represented by musculoskeletal injuries, while the most dangerous and deleterious is sudden cardiac death. Intense physical activity does raise a small risk of cardiac death, particularly for sedentary persons with a genetic predisposition for sudden death and in athletes with underlying cardiopathy, such as silent ischemic heart disease. Nonetheless, the longer term reduction in overall death risk from regular exercise outweighs any minute potential for acute cardiovascular complications. Physical activity has beneficial effects in all sectors of life, enhancing cardiac, pulmonary and muscular function. Therefore physical activity must be encouraged from the early years of life mainly in the young, however the effects of physical exercise on the cardiovascular system, when it is very competitive, may be dangerous. Strenuous exercise can also result "paradoxically" harmful in time. For this reason the preparticipation screening program of athletes has the goal of the early identification of previously unsuspected cardiovascular disease and the disqualification of the athletes in the hope that these strategies will reduce the incidence of sudden cardiac death. Screening participation in order to discover early stages of malignant neoplasia (e.g. breast and colon cancer) in asymptomatic stage and thus prevent reaching final stages of the disease has been widely accepted. Vice versa, although atherosclerotic cardiovascular disease causes more deaths and disabilities than all the causes of death correlated to cancer, there are no precise guidelines concerning the screening of asymptomatic elements suffering from atherosclerosis, and even fewer recommendations, apart from the recent Shape [37] program, which presents practical recommendations concerning cardiovascular screening for asymptomatic people at cardiovascular risk. Shape guidelines propose screening via non-invasive investigation for all asymptomatic males aged between 45 and 75 years, and for all asymptomatic females between the ages of 55 and 75 (except those persons clearly defined as being low-risk), in order to discover and

6

treat those subjects struck by sub-clinical atherosclerosis. Coronary atherosclerosis is the main cause of death in developed countries and is becoming the main cause of death in the rest of the world too [79] [75]. However, many patients with predictable coronary disease are asymptomatic [80]. As is well-known, clinically significant coronary atherosclerosis is uncommon in subjects, particularly males, under 40 years of age and in pre-menopause females, but the risk grows as age increases and also in the presence of factors of classic risks such as smoking, hypertension, diabetes, hypercholesterolemia, and ischemic heart disease familiarity. Silent myocardial ischemia is, by definition, present in asymptomatic subjects, and particularly in those subjects who present underlying factors of cardiovascular risk. Silent myocardial ischemia is a major component of the total ischemic burden for patients with coronary artery disease (CAD); it is estimated that between 2 and 3 million persons with stable CAD have evidence of silent ischemia. This is very important for those doctors who have to identify the existence of silent ischemic cardiopathy in consideration of the fact that this situation is predictive of an increase in the risk of even fatal, cardiac events [54]. In studies, albeit not recent, which assessed a broad spectrum of the population, the prevalence of silent ischemic cardiopathy was esteemed at around 4 – 4,5% in middle-aged men (in their fifties) with accompanying asymptomatic coronary heart disease and the presence of myocardial ischemia evoked by exercise stress test on the tread-mill [78] [34]. Consequently, there has been great interest in recent years in developing screening strategies through which severe asymptomatic coronary heart disease could be diagnosed prematurely [47]. Coronary disease can be considered an 'iceberg' where a small part of the subjects are symptomatic for angina pectoris, whilst the majority of individuals suffering from coronary heart disease have no symptoms at all [21]. The most common symptom in ischemic heart disease to appear first, is angina pectoris, due to coronary atherosclerosis, although in a few subjects the first sign may be myocardial infarction, or even, sudden death [98]. It has been calculated that from one to two million middle aged males in the United States of America (i.e. around 5% of the population) are suffering from asymptomatic coronary heart disease, also known as, "silent myocardial ischemia" [98]. Myocardial ischemia, be it silent or asymptomatic, is defined as an objective documentation of myocardial ischemia, in the absence of angina or its equivalents [18]. Among the subjects who can be asymptomatic coronary heart disease carriers, athletes also come into this category, i.e. individuals who regularly practice and compete in sports events at highly competitive athletic levels. Most of the patients with silent myocardial ischemia due to coronary artery disease are athletes. It is important for physicians to know that the most common symptom as myocardial ischemia is the absence of symptoms. Silent myocardial ischemia is not the same as silent coronary artery disease. Symptomatic angina is the tip of the ischemic iceberg and in athletes is smaller than non -athletes. Athletes change their perception of ischemic stimulus and increasing pain threshold from increased circulating endorphin levels. Silent myocardial ischemia is more prevalent than angina in patients with coronary artery disease, and athletes are not immune to this disease. As atherosclerosis disease is an evolutive, degenerative process, as well as being inflammatory, increasing and worsening as time passes, it is clear that older individuals, thus, athletes too, have a higher probability of running or cycling with underlying silent ischemic coronary heart disease [57]. Athletes are normally considered individuals in good if not great health, thus when one of them is struck by sudden death, it creates uproar and consternation. However, just as what happens among the population on a whole, athletes can harbour unrecognized cardiac diseases, just like asymptomatic atherosclerotic coronary heart disease, or congenital abnormalities which can place them in the sights of high risk sudden death [90]. Competitive sport at high cardiovascular impact is dangerous for fatal arrhythmia in subjects predisposed to and suffering from coronary atherosclerosis disease [10].

Male athletes are hit by coronary artery disease much more than female athletes (at a rate of 10 to1). This can be attributed to the fact that more male athletes take part in competitive sports and there is also a tendency to greater intensity in the training of male athletes. The male sex is in itself a risk factor in coronary heart disease, and that is because of the higher rate of cardiac abnormalities and premature atherosclerotic coronary heart disease in male athletes as opposed to females [22]. The paradox is that whilst a lack of physical activity in time has been correlated to an increase in the negative effects on health including the development of coronary heart disease, obesity and global increase in deaths, the practice of regular physical activity has clearly demonstrated the prevention and retarding in the advancement of coronary heart disease, however vigorous physical exercise in individuals over 40 is also associated with an increase in the risk of sudden death and myocardial infarction [100-101]. Even though the advantages and benefits gained through the practice of physical exercise exceed the risks connected to it, athletes of a certain age are warned and encouraged to undergo accurate medical screening in order to identify any problem of a cardiac nature before participating in competitive sport activities [68]. Athlete screening strategies [30] around the world vary widely, and some athletes are never screened with a preparticipation physical evaluation. In Italy the structure of a sports preparticipation screening include: (1) history with or without a structured questionaire and physical exam; ECG, exercise ECG stress testing, urinalysis, and spirometry, and other specific test for particular sports. Exam intervals vary from 1 to 2 years. The sports preparticipation screening is more than a "heart" exam [90], although the main cause for exclusion from competitive sport is almost always caused by heart disease. However, there are other reasons for carrying it out, including its potential use as a tool in reducing sport injury risks, counseling for high-risk behaviors, screening for chronic disease including depression, and placing an athlete face-to-face with a physician or other health care provider.

Investigation methods and accurate screening tests for Ischemic Coronary Disease

There are two complementary methods of screening, qualified to reduce morbidity and mortality in coronary atherosclerosis. The first includes the assessment and correction of modifiable factors of cardiac risk, such as hypertension, hypercholesterolemia, smoking, physical inactivity and diet. The second strategy is represented by early diagnosis of asymptomatic coronary heart disease, for which in the last 10 to 15 years there has been development in the techniques through which an important but asymptomatic coronary heart disease can be diagnosed [47]. The electrocardiography remains the most widely used instrument for discovering myocardial ischemia [25-26]. Amongst the main tests for diagnosing silent coronary sclerosis are electrocardiograms (ECG), at rest and above all during maximum effort , which can furnish the evidence of a silent, progressive myocardial infarction or of an asymptomatic cardiac ischemia [47].

The assessment of the prevalence of silent myocardial ischemia in the general population comes from studies that engaged electrocardiographic monitoring during exercise stress tests, such as, for example, the participants in the Seattle Heart Watch [14] study or the Lipid Research Clinics Program study, who were individuals chosen amongst the 'normal' population, apparently symptomless and having first undergone stress tests and consequently follow-up in order to investigate the relevance of the electrographic alternations of silent ischemia. The results of the two studies drew attention to the fact that out of 10.000 asymptomatic subjects studied, 500 (5%) had an abnormal stress test, 50% of these individuals resulted in having coronary heart disease on coronary angiography.

Can a maximal exercise stress testing with electrocardiographic monitoring therefore, improve the diagnostic capacities, predictive of future coronary events, in asymptomatic individuals?

Some studies [55] have demonstrated that a ST segment depression with horizontal or descending pattern $> 0 =$ to 1mm in evoked by stress test is a strong predictor of future coronary events, those like angina pectoris, myocardial infarction, and even, sudden death. Epson and collaborators [32] put the results of Bruce's and Erikksen's [35] studies together in order to estimate that in 10.000 asymptomatic individuals tested, 500 (5%) demonstrated an abnormal stress test result, 50% of these individuals showing angiographic signs of coronary heart disease. In these individuals there was a 0,7% annual incidence of coronary events, in contrast with the 0,06% in annual deaths that take place in individuals with a negative stress test. In the follow up registered in the Lipid Research Clinics study [31], the asymptomatic individuals with positive stress tests had a cardiovascular mortality increase five times superior, indicating that the electrocardiographic evidence of ischemia is therefore an independent predictive factor of mortality.

Other studies showed that the presence of silent myocardial ischemia in the exercise stress test has predictive value in cardiovascular events of the angina type rather than myocardial infarction or death and the coexistence of a conventional risk factor together with the electrocardiographic signs of ST segment depression, substantially increases the realistic risk of coronary heart disease events [65 98]. Various alterations in the ECG at rest (ST segment depression, Inversion of the T wave, Q waves and deviation of the cardiac axis) are related to an increased probability of coronary heart disease atherosclerosis and future cardiac events. However these findings are not frequent in asymptomatic individuals, as they only concern 1- 4% of middle-aged male individuals who have no clinical signs of coronary heart disease [87 94] and are not specific to this kind of illness. About a third or a half of asymptomatic patients with coronaries angiographically undamaged, in the resting ECG presents Q waves, inversion of T waves or changes in the ST-T segment, whilst an altogether normal ECG does not exclude coronary atherosclerosis. The asymptomatic individuals with basic ECG (Q waves, ST segment depression, T wave inversion, left ventricular hypertrophy and premature ventricular contractions) are however more at risk from future coronary heart disease events [87]. An ECG carried out under stress is definitely more accurate than one at rest to diagnose clinically important coronary heart disease atherosclerosis, and the variations in the ECG are often

11

not manifest until the atherosclerosis plaques have advanced to such a state that coronary flow is significantly impeded [33].

The majority of asymptomatic individuals with abnormalities in the ECG tracing under stress (generally defined by a specific value of the ST segment depression) do not present basic coronary heart disease [26]. Several situations are responsible for causing a depression in the ST segment during physical effort in absence of a significant obstruction in one of the main coronary arteries. Any lesion in cardiac mechanics that creates left ventricular overloading and increased needs, such as e.g. a mitral valve or aortic dysfunction, pulmonary hypertension, left ventricular hypertrophy, as well as a relative coronary insufficiency, are no doubt the main causes of false positive stress tests relative to the ST segment depression in individuals with increased left ventricular mass [93]. Ulterior studies confirm that maximal stress test is commonly considered a potentiality in early diagnosis of ischemic coronary heart disease [47-85], because it is simple to carry out, inexpensive and accurate [45-87]. Nevertheless, low precision and in accuracy of the stress ECG in diagnosing hemodynamically significant coronary stenosis, even in asymptomatic individuals, has brought about recommendations not to use the stress test as a screening instrument, as well in the USPSTF [43] report which recalls Guidelines on stress tests elaborated by ACC/AHA in 2002 [2], which specify that the sensitivity and specific nature of the stress test are inversely correlated according to the elements tested from which a diverse prognostic assessment evolves, as is reported in the latest European guidelines on cardiovascular prevention which clearly and totally place the significance of the stress test together with the pre-test probability of disease.

Some meta analysis studied variability in the diagnostic accuracy of the stress test and indicated a wide variability in sensitivity (average value 68%, with a wide range from 23 - 100% and a 16% Standard Deviation - SD),and in specificity (with an average value of 77%, ranging from 17 – 100% and a DS of 17%). These recommendations are largely based on many publications documenting the limitations in the modifications of the ST segment in the diagnosis of ischemic coronary heart disease in asymptomatic individuals. In fact, when the maximum stress test is simply used as a diagnostic test it is advisable to be aware that false positive tests are common amongst asymptomatic adult individuals, especially females, and that could determine further unnecessary investigation, useless treatment, disease labelling [43]. F. Pigozzi and colleagues published a study [84] on the role of the stress test in athletes, the conclusion of which affirms the discovery of a ST segment depression during the stress test of these individuals when unaccompanied by symptoms and/or complex ventricular arrhythmia. With further imaging, such as myocardial scintigraphy, or negative echo-stress, should not be held as cardiac re-modelling on a physiological basis induced by strain.

However, Rywik and coworkers [88] have established that depression of the ST segment that appears in the active recovery period of the stress test, in apparently asymptomatic individuals, represents an adverse prognosis event, similar to the importance of the ST depression in the course of the exercise. Rywik et al. [88] as already indicated, attach independent prognostic significance for future cardiovascular events in asymptomatic individuals to the ischemic modifications in the ST segment during the stress test and an intensification of the preceding anomalies of the right ventricular (ST segment depression over 1mm) at rest.

It is also interesting to notice that the presence (or lack of) chest pain in diabetic patients with foregoing vascular events and therefore with a high probability of disease, who present an ischemic response due to stress, obtained once again from the ST depression does not modify the prognosis concerning the risk of running into cardiac events in the following 2 years, as demonstrated by Callaham et al [15]. The significance of the quantitative assessment of the ST depression has been studied by Kaul and collaborators [58], who found that the ST segment depression $> 0 =$ up to 2 mm was a marker of high risk for acute coronary syndrome.

Shlom Stern [92] affirms that the quantitative value in the ST segment as the measure of the level of myocardial ischemia is still far from being absolutely clear, not only in the level of exercise carried out requested for the development of the ischemia, but also profundity and duration,

the number of cardiac derivations in which it appears, and furthermore, the presence or absence of T-wave, are equally important factors in diagnosis and prognosis [92].

Furthermore, the interpretation of the data in the modifications of the ST segment, plus the consideration of the relative analysis not only of the T segment but the stress test prognostic assessment rather than only a diagnostic one [64], suggests that the former could be underestimated, in the sense that the positive significance of the stress test and anomalies induced by it are not always wholly understood and well assessed.

Thallium-201 [28 97], the stress echocardiography or pharmaceutically induced stress and dynamic electrocardiography (with Holter monitoring) are less used as screening methods.

The efficacy of each of these screening tests can be estimated on the basis of (a) the test's capacity in diagnosing the presence of atherosclerotic plaque and (b) the capacity to foresee the onset of an important clinical event in the future (acute myocardial infarction, sudden death).

The addition of Thallium-201 scintigraphy to conventional stress tests improves the accuracy of the latter in diagnosing coronary atherosclerosis, making it a useful diagnostic test for individuals with coronary heart disease symptoms [62 28]. Due to these limits and its costs, Thallium-201 scintigraphy is not considered an optimum method of screening for asymptomatic individuals [39]. To clarify the significance of angina during a stress scintigraphy with ischemic type anomalies of the distribution of Thallium, Heller and colleagues [50], studied 129 patients with anomalies of this kind and angina, which were compared to 105 patients, with the same scintigraphic alterations, but no angina (silent ischemia). During 62 months of follow up, no survival differences appeared. The authors, thus, decided that silent ischemia identified through the stress scintigraphy had the same unfavourable prognostic implications as ischemia associated with angina.

The association between stress ECG and myocardial scintigraphy with Thallium-201 seems a more accurate method than a simple stress ECG in order to predict future coronary heart disease events in apparently healthy individuals, as a positive concordance in the two tests revealed a probability of suffering a coronary event 3,6 times superior to those individuals whose tests did not match [39]. All things considered, the importance of silent ischemia in asymptomatic individuals has been confirmed by the studies of Droste and colleagues [29], who showed that absolutely asymptomatic coronary heart disease patients with stress test have a higher mortality rate (over a 12 year follow-up period) than the general population of the same age.

Biagini et al. [12], more recently published, an observational study in 'Heart' on the long term outcomes of individuals divided into asymptomatic and symptomatic, who had signs of silent ischemia, on carrying out stress test with dobutamine , drew the same conclusions [13].

1st Level Sport Medicine Assessment of a Master Athlete (35 or over in age)

professional competitor

The most numerous group of asymptomatic individuals in Italy who have to undergo stress tests is composed of individuals who practice sports at a competitive level and are obliged by law, in order to safeguard public health [81], to carry out a medical check-up annually.

To this effect in order to assess fitness, specific cardiological protocols have been created when concerning any suspicion of silent ischemic coronary heart disease and therefore, in the presence of electrocardiographic anomalies in ventricular polarization, whether at rest or under stress, without any proven documented morphological cardiac alternations, recommend further investigation, especially in sports people in the $> 35 - 40$ age group [90].

Master athletes represent an ever increasing number, in the micro-cosmos of the athletic world, which includes various sports, above all those tough sports which really engage the cardio-circulatory system, like cycling, marathon running, triathlon, thus absolutely requiring a medical check-up, in order to exclude the presence of silent ischemic coronary heart disease, in any of these individuals [68-81-82].

Even though everyone thinks of a competitive athlete as being in great health and therefore 'immune' from cardiac pathologies, a relationship has been observed for some time, between vigorous, physical activity and sudden death in Master athletes, in the presence of underlying cardiological disease [67].

Epidemiological data suggests that such events occur more in Master athletes as opposed to younger ones, at a risk estimated around 1/15000 to 1/18000 in young athletes to around 1/100.000 to 1/300.000 in Masters [66].

The principal cause of death, in Master athletes, is coronary heart disease, which, on the basis of autopsy studies, usually consists in severe obstruction of the coronary lumen, caused by atherosclerotic plaque, in one or more of the principal coronary arteries [77-86].

The two main mechanisms determining sudden death related to physical exercise are; coronary spasm and plaque break-up [9-80].

In fact, although physical exercise dilates normal coronary arteries, it can induce spasm in coronaries struck by atherosclerosis plaques with significant narrowing, or determine the breakage of plaque and consequently, a thrombotic event [91].

Finally, myocardial ischemia brought on by physical exercise can provoke fatal arrhythmias like ventricular fibrillation [33-67], even in individuals with atherosclerotic lesions not considered critical (with narrowing superior to 50 – 60 %of the coronary lumen).

Recent evidence too, has shown the high incidence of silent ischemic coronary heart disease brought on by exercise, and specifically by the stress test undertaken by Master athletes [57].

In fact, it emerges, from this study that, contrary to what was believed, the prevalence of an asymptomatic ST segment depression, at maximal stress testing was absolutely identical in tested individuals, whether Master athletes or males leading sedentary lives [55].

The authors concluded that the presence of the allele of apoliprotein E4 in Master athletes was correlated to increased risk in developing ischemic alterations of the myocardium during maximal exercise stress tests [58].

In Master athletes who voluntarily refrained from training for a three-month period and in follow-up, the presence of myocardial ischemia induced by maximal stress test, carried out at the end of inactivity was correlated to a greater incidence of negative cardiac events (sudden death, coronary aorta by-pass) in the follow up period [11].

Other observations suggest that sudden death and the occurrence of cardiac events such as myocardial infarction in fact aren't rare in Master athletes [16 71 86 101].

The main aim in the cardiovascular screening of competitive athletes is to identify those individuals with unsuspected coronary heart disease and interrupt any training and competitive events so as to minimize the risks of their suffering sudden death on the sports field, whether it be in practice or during competitions [67]. Therefore, the screening tests and protocols used in the exercise stress testing should be specially directed to discovering any possible silent ischemic coronary heart disease, in Master athletes [25 26 41 5361].

These individuals definitely represent a low-risk group, as the majority of them do not present the factors of risk, such as, smoking, hypertension, obesity, dyslipidemia and obviously, a sedentary life-style, but even all that does not exclude the presence of silent ischemic coronary heart disease, with resulting negative prognosis. Existing data (not recent) suggests a high rate of false positive tests in athletes as opposed to sedentary life style individuals [84].

Hood and Northcote [53], for example, reported a 15,8 % in an ST segment depression falsely positive, in highly trained veteran endurance athletes.

Katzel et al.[57], as well, found a 13 % ST segment depression, in Master athletes with no evidence of coronary heart disease, just as Pigozzi and colleagues, whose studies revealed false ST segment depression in 2,6 % of the athletes who underwent testing, and no false ST segment depression in sedentary subjects. One can derive from the above that present recommendations on the usefulness of stress tests in general, such as screenings and early diagnosis of cardiovascular disease are varied and in disagreement.

For example, routine ECG at rest as a screening test for coronary artery disease in asymptomatic adults is neither advised by the American College of Physicians (ACP) [30] nor by the Canadian Task Force in their Health Organization Procedure [16].

The American Academy of Family Physicians (AAFP) recommends a basic ECG for males aged 40 and over, with two or more cardiovascular factors of risk, and for males leading sedentary life styles the recommendation is under assessment [5].

A task force sponsored by the American College of Cardiology and American Heart Association (ACC/AHA) advises a basic check up for all people over 40 and those about to undertake stress tests [6].

The American College of Sports Medicine advises, prior to undertaking intense physical activity, undergoing a stress test in males aged forty and over (therefore presumably a good idea for Master Athletes), and in females over fifty, as well as asymptomatic individuals with multiple cardiac risk factors [7].

More recently recommendations have been put together for early screening at competitions through assessment and ascertainment of possible cardiovascular pathologies in Master athletes [68] that foresee specific guide lines so that adequate cardiovascular assessment be finalized for the identification of individuals suffering from underlying cardiovascular disease, and above all for revealing silent ischemic heart disease, prior to commencing any training program and to guarantee and safeguard health and safety in athletes over forty years of age[26].

In agreement with guidelines published in 2001 by World Health Federation (WHF), International Federation of Sports Medicine and the AHA [68], screening carried out by ECG monitoring during maximal stress testing should be used in assessing males over 40 – 50 and or,women over 50 – 55 with an independent factor of coronary risk (such as hypercholesterolemia or dyslipidemia, arterial hypertension, low levels of HDL cholesterol, the habit of smoking, and mellitus diabetes) or a history of myocardial infarction or sudden death in first level family members under sixty years of age. The same test, furthermore, is recommended for all Master Athletes of any age with suggestive symptoms for coronary heart disease and all athletes over [65].

In the result of positivity, the guidelines mentioned, recommend carrying out further tests for complete diagnosis. It is therefore reasonable to combine the stress test with diagnostic imaging (myocardial scan in perfusion or stress echocardiogram) in those athletes who present significant electrocardiographic anomalies. Finally, recent recommendations [82] regarding participation in highly competitive sports of athletes with cardiovascular disease confirm a prevalence of ischemic coronary heart disease in individuals aged over 35, advising competing Master athletes with signs of silent or symptomatic ischemic coronary heart disease, or rather when unequivocal signs of myocardial ischemia induced by stress test emerge, to have coronary angiography vital in precisely assessing possible and significant haemodynamic obstructions in the blood flow.

These recommendations indicate furthermore a high probability of adverse cardiac events induced by strenuous effort, when at least one or more of the following criteria are present:

- echocardiographic or scintigraphic evidence of a left ventricular ejection fraction < 50 %;
- ischemia brought on by stress (with ST segment depression > 1 mm in at least two derivations) at stress test,
- presence of dyspnoea (ergo equivalent angina) or syncope;
- appearance of frequent , complex ventricular arrhythmia at rest or during exercise stress test;
- evidence of significant narrowing in a major coronary artery (over 70 %) or stenosis (over 50 %) of left principal coronary artery.

In conclusion, the authorities affirm that silent cardiac ischemia increases the risk of cardiac arrest during physical exercise induced by stress in the same way as individuals with symptomatic ischemic heart disease [32-33].

Personal Cases: experiences and management of silent ischemia cardiopathy of a

primary level Sport medicine Centre Survey.

The objective of this thesis in presenting 10 clinical cases relative to the 1st level in highly competitive Master athletes, practicing endurance sports sets its sights on illustrating the clinical procedure and follow-up, that ensues the electrocardiographic evidence characterized by significant depression and therefore pathological of the ST segment and relative parameters in Master athletes through the maximal test on specific ergometer and with ad hoc protocol.

As is well known myocardial ischemia can appear in three classic modifications of the ST segment in the surface ECG, such as depression, elevation and normalization.

The ST segment depression is the most common manifestation of myocardial ischemia, caused by stress effort, and therefore is thus the most widely used electrocardiograph criteria of immediate visible comparison and therefore easily traceable during the maximum test through continuous monitoring with ad hoc oscilloscope [25].

It usually reflects a widespread subendocardial ischemia, the direction of the carrier is largely determined by the ischemic area and the position of the heart in the (thoracic) chest.

The standard criteria used by the author, and widely accepted for an abnormal ultrasound response is the horizontal or down sloping_ of the ST segment depression of 0,10 mV (1,0 mm) that remain after 80 ms from point J, in more than one electrocardiographic lead initially isoelectric and in at least three consecutive heart beats [41].

Morphologically, the aspect of the ST segment depression can be extremely variable, however the patterns of surely positive when the ST segment depression are of the following types:

- descending/down sloping

  b) horizontal or square

  c) slow ascending

(increased ST depression of point J by 1 mm, at a rate Qx/Qt >0,5) [70] [46]

The PR segment is the reference point with which the following segment QT is compared.

A down sloping ST depression, is indicative of greater ischemia compared with the pattern of horizontal or slow ascending type.

Usually a 'quickly ascending' pattern of ST segment depression is not considered pathological in which the rate Qx/Qt < 0,5, even if point J is more than 1 mm in depression, and the author of this manuscript in complete agreement with other authors [96] feels that the 1,5 mm depression at 80 ms after point J is the most reasonable criteria for a positive result.

The assessment was however polyparametric in order to increase diagnostic accuracy as suggested by Kligfield [61], and included the calculation of the ST/HR slope or ST/HR index, that is, the adjustments of the depression in the QT segment compared to cardiac frequency and the relative index and,'ad abundantiam, the assessment of the R wave width in the V5 lead, even if in everyday situations ulterior factors correlated to the probability and the severity of the coronary illness include, level, data, persistence during the stage of recovery and the number of leads that present ST segment depression. [73]

The total number of screened athletes (see Statistics report) in these 5 years is 1958 (3109 examinations), composed by 1250 (66%) < 40 in age and 648 (34%) aged > 40 (Master athletes) 1898 athletes were suitable (97%), whilst the unsuitable subjects were 37 (1,95%), with the remaining 23 (1,2%) not taken into consideration.

The percentage of unsuitable athletes over 40 was the same at 3,86%, whilst in athletes under 40 considered unsuitable it was 0,96%.

The causes of unsuitability in Master athletes were all of a cardiac nature, including 7 (28%) due to silent ischemic cardiopathy, whilst the remaining ones were equally divided into, arrhythmic, mostly ventricular, valvulopathies and severe arterial hypertension.

Among the athletes who suffered from silent or asymptomatic ischemic heart disease, 4 (57%)) had already been revascularized with coronary artery bypass grafting (CABG) and stenting. .

Amongst the suspended athletes another five individuals had anomalies of ventricular repolarization suggesting myocardial ischemia brought on by stress effort, but for various motives they continued the required diagnostic protocol with secondary level control (myocardial scintigraphy) and were archived for incomplete documentation.

Ten clinical cases are to follow, with significant anomalies in vascular repolarization, suggesting myocardial infarction brought on by stress effort, found during an ergometric exercise test, in the course of a test on a cycle ergometer or treadmill whilst testing for annual check-up for competitive sports carried out in the author's sport medicine surgery, in a 5-year period going from the beginning of 2002 to the end of 2006.

The clinical protocol carried out, the signs of significant depression in the ST segment following above mentioned criteria, and sub-division of cases into categories, true positive and false positive on the basis of the results of coronary angiography in nine individuals and in one case, from a computed tomography (CT) coronary angiography, considered still today, the 'Gold Standard' exam, in coronary atherosclerosis and ischemic heart disease is here described.

The clinical cases concerning competitive Master athletes (aged over 40), of which five, amateur marathon runners and the other five, professional cyclists, taking part in medium-long length racing competitions.

All the athletes who were examined, underwent maximal exercise testing, aimed at, reaching and overcoming anaerobic threshold on specific ergometer with the electrocardiographic monitoring of 6 - 12 leads on monitor and documenting all leads at every rising step as well as in the period of immediate recovery.

These individuals were oriented towards secondary level exams (exercise stress testing with myocardial scintigraphy or stress echocardiography) and third level cardiological ones (invasive or non invasive CT coronary angiography).

Five individuals out of seven resulted true positive, myocardial revascularization took place for critically severe coronary heart disease, mono or multivessel disease and in one case including critical stenosis of the left coronary common trunk.

	Totale	< 40 anni	>= 40 anni
Atleti idonei	1898	1250	648
Atleti non idonei	37	12	25
Atleti sospesi	23	4	19

Totale Visite Mediche Effettuate   **3109**

Totale Atleti Visitati   **1958**

Totale Visite Effettuate

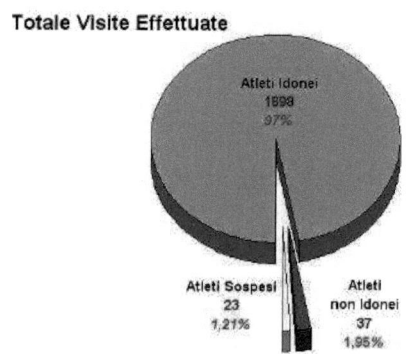

Atleti Idonei
1899
97%

Atleti Sospesi
23
1,21%

Atleti
non Idonei
37
1,95%

Totale = total

> < 40 anni = > < 40 yrs old

Atleti idonei = Suitable fit athletes

Atleti non idonei = Unsuitable unfit Athletes

Totale Visite Mediche effettuate, Totale Visite effettuate = Total number of examinations carried out

Totale Atleti Visitati = Total number of athletes examined

Atleti idonei = Fit athletes

24

Atleti sospesi	= Suspended athletes
Athleti non idonei	= Unfit Athletes
Sotto i 40 anni	= Under 40 yrs old
Sopra i 40 anni	= Over 40 yrs old

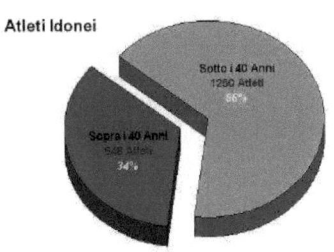

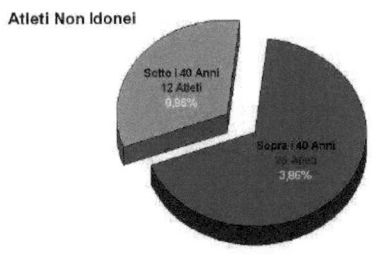

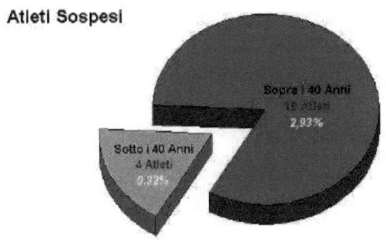

TRUE POSITIVES

Case 1 D.E. (Amateur, Marathon runner aged 59) Critical stenosis of common trunk.

In January 2002 the athlete underwent a fitness examination specific to track and field events, for

his annual check-up, which he regularly carried out at the author's Sport Medicine Centre.

The athlete had been seen through the years and had always obtained his eligibility certificate

permitting him to do competitive sport.

His medical history was positive for hypercholesterolemia, which not had been treated pharmacologically,

while familiarity was doubtful for ischemic heart disease.

In fact, the athlete complained of bilateral tinnitus and reported continuous use of hypno-inducers.

Nothing particularly significant was relevant in his basic ECG, so maximal exercise stress testing

on the treadmill was carried out, following the Astrand protocol, for advanced walkers (keeping up

a constant speed of 13 km/h, after 5 km warm up at 4 Km/h and 0 % slope, increasing 3,5 % every

2 min until reaching muscular exhaustion.

The test was interrupted at heart rate of 166 bpm (> 100% theoretical maximal heart rate), at a level

of 12,5 Metabolic Equivalents (METS), both from muscular exhaustion and by the appearance of

down-sloping depression of the ST segment of 3–4 mm at 80ms after the J point in the precordial

deviations from V3 to V6.

The anomalous pattern of the ST segment was observed as being present up to 6-9th minute of

active recovery with a gradual but slow restoring of normal, ventricular repolarization.

The subject was absolutely asymptomatic for the whole duration of the test.

The appearance of the electrocardiograph tracing resulted clearly modified in respect to those of the

preceding years, which had always been negative.

At this point a TL201 myocardial scintigraphy with maximal stress effort by cycloergometer test,

was requested, and carried out on 22nd Feb 2002, also showing significant electrocardiographic aspects for ST segment depression in V4-V6 at 175 watts extended charge, with return to basic aspect after more than 5 min recovery time.

The perfusional scintigraphy showed clear evidence of hypocaptation in the tracing, moderate and reversible on behalf of the anterior-septal, inferior and of inferior lateral wall.

The conclusions were exam results compatible with inducible exercise myocardial ischemia, at high work load, involving the anterior septal inferior, infero lateral wall.

Despite this unequivocal evidence there was a certain delay, determined by the scarce conviction of the referring cardiologist, before deciding on the coronography, which showed critical ostial stenosis of the common trunk with conserved systolic function of the left ventricular.

On 31st May 2002 the patient was operated for myocardial revascularization via Coronary Artery Bypass Graft surgery (CABG) with LIMA on DA and RIMA on MO). The patient, has been in great health since then and practices walking, at amateur level.

Case N° 2 P.P (amateur cycling competitor, aged 43) Non critical bivascular coronoropathy.

In December 2002, a 43 yr old cyclist, positive for coronary artery disease (CAD) familiarity (father died from dilated cardio myopathy on ischemic basis and a brother suffering from stable angina) underwent a sport medical examination for a fitness certificate in cycling.

Heavy smoking was considered a major risk factor in the patient's case history.

 A preceding medical examination undergone by the cyclist in the author's surgery in 1993 had indicated nothing pathological, nor did anything result from further fitness tests carried out elsewhere. On 23rd December, the 43 year old underwent a basal ECG with normal results.

He was, therefore, given a normal exercise stress testing on the cycloergometer with protocol increasing at 25 watt every 90 sec after adequate warm up.

From the 6th minute of exercise, 1 mm anomalies in the ventricular repolarization (VR) appeared in reference to line Q-Q and PR segment, the test was interrupted at the 10th minute for rigidity and upward sloping slow depression with horizontal pattern of the ST segment by over 2 mm in the deviations from V3 to V6 (see fig. 2).

The anomaly of the ST segment slowly receded even if at the 3rd minute of active recovery a 1mm ST depression was still evident.

The athlete had no symptoms throughout the test, at all.

On 19th December 2002 the subject underwent a professional myocardial scintigraphy with TL201, before and after stress testing exercise at the cyclo-ergometer carried out at the Nuclear Medicine Department of Cesena Hospital with measuring 25 watt protocol every 2 minutes up to 250 watts. The test was interrupted, due to muscular exhaustion at 98% of Maximal heart rate and a Double Product (DP) = 34.600. **No** electrocardiographic alterations were registered, however, of the ventricular repolarization (see fig.1). The myocardial scintigraphy revealed however, a light myocardial hyperfusion from maximal stress effort to high workload.

The certificate of fitness, just for precaution, was not given because of the athlete's refusal, ill-advised by his own general practitioner, to undergo a coronary angiography

I consequently found out that the athlete in the year 2003, had again undergone a stress ECG, in a cardiological structure and had had negative results. The following year 2004, the cyclist again underwent a maximal exercise stress testing at a cardiological centre and that time got a positive result; in 2005, following perfusional myocardial scintigraphy with TL201 which resulted positive for a light hypoperfusion at high work load at the inferior septal and with signs of 40% ejection fraction (EF) and 43% after effort. Consequently study of coronary angiography, which showed signs of coronary atherosclerotic calcification above all in the anterior branch of the proximal segment with mild to moderate stenosis, eccentric and segmentary, in the whole of the first segment although not haemodynamically significant; critical stenosis of a septal branch. Due to his young age, the familiarity and the hypercholesterolomy, his referring cardiologists decided upon pharmaceutical therapy and haemodynamic check-up. A year onward, the cyclist continues his

sporting activity. Fig. 1

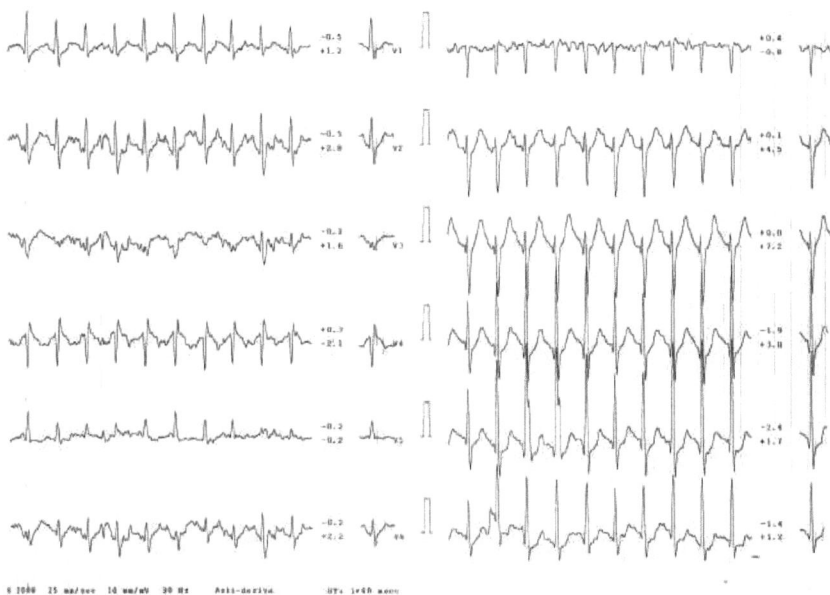

Fig. 2

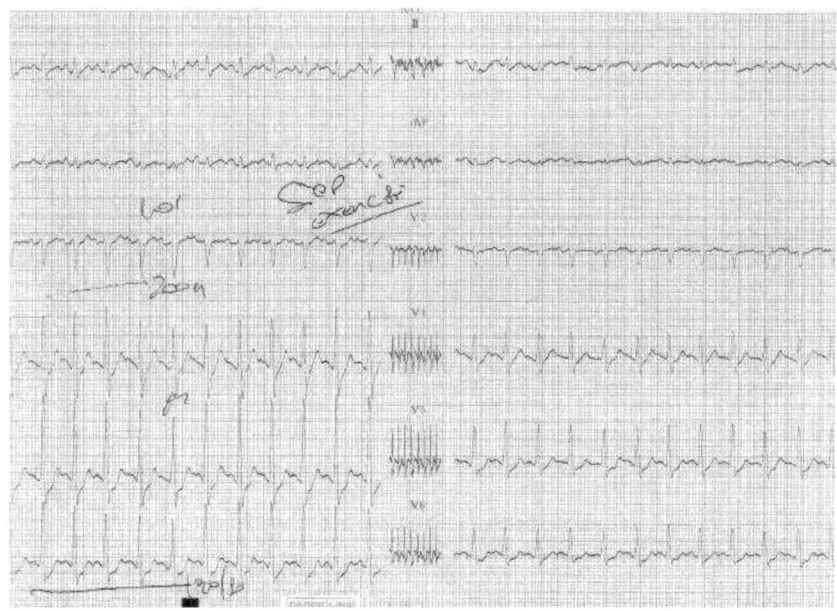

Case 3 B.P. (advanced Fiidal amateur runner aged 46) with critical coronaropathy in proximal descending artery (DA) and ostial stenosis of the first diagonal branch.

Amateur athlete with positive familiarity of case history for ischemic cardiopathy (father, brother), had always had positive results in preceding years when undergoing fitness tests for track-and-field athletes and walkers. Light to moderate smoking, that is, around 10 cigarettes daily, was amongst the classic risk factors. On Feb. 14th 2005, the athlete underwent a sports pre-participation screening.

Resting ECG indicated sinusal bradycardia with right bundle branch block and aspecific anomalies of ventricular repolarization.

The following stress exercise testing on the cyclo-ergometer (preferred to the tread-mill for lengthening of femoral biceps), was interrupted because of the presence of anomalies of the ventricular repolarization (AVR) (i.e. ST segment depression from V4a to V4 for about 4 mm) with horizontal and down-sloping pattern, that began at the 10th minute of testing, (see fig. 4)

These anomalies of VR, which were ischemic, gradually disappeared during the period of active recovery. The individual had remained absolutely asymptomatic throughout the test.

On March 3rd 2005, he underwent a myocardial scintigraphy with TL201, with maximal stress test on the cyclo-ergometer.

On that occasion the ECG stress test did **NOT** indicate any anomalies of the VR (see fig. 3) whilst the perfusional scintigraphy indicated a light and reversible hypocaptation of the interventricular septum. A study of the global, regional and volumetric functioning of the left ventricular however indicated a post stress ejection fraction equal to 52%, reason for which the cardiologist decided on a compatible exam with light myocardial hypoperfusion from stress effort high workload involving the intra ventricular septum.

However, the athlete underwent a coronary angiography, on 12th May 2005, which indicated an obstruction in the proximal segment of the anterior diagonal branch.

This was later followed by myocardial revascularization via PTCA and placement of drug medical stent on IVA +PTCA on the ostium of the first diagonal branch.

In 2006 the veteran runner was examined again and assessed for fitness in competition, which he passed at the end of his sport medicine examination with no indication of anomalies in the VR, negative results for reduced coronary reserves and excellent cardio-circulatory efficiency.

In fact the 2003 COCIS affirms that in subjects with isolated stenosis and favourable angioplasty for efficient recanalization, after at least a year from procedure, fitness for sports activity, with medium to high cardio circulatory demands, can be taken into consideration, obviously respecting the necessary 6 month – checkups.

Fig 3

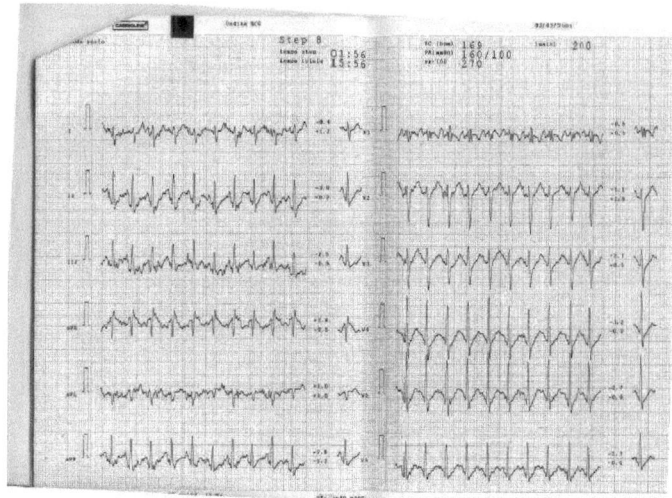

Fig 4

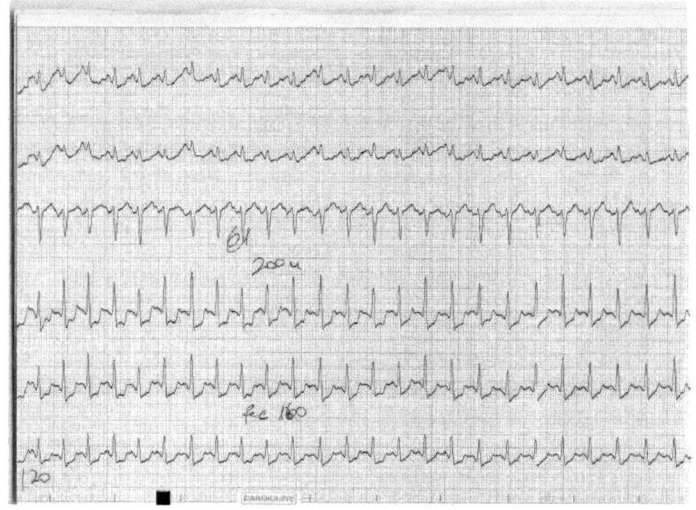

Case 4 V.O. (67 years old amateur cyclist) critical multi-vessel coronary artery disease treated firstly by myocardial revascularization via Percutaneous Transluminal Coronary Angioplasty (PTCA) and then by CABG.

Competitive athlete who requested fitness certificate for competitive cycling in January 2005 in order to resolve a diagnostic doubt relative to asymptomatic anomalies of ventricular repolarization present in preceding fitness tests carried out elsewhere.

Other secondary level cardiological tests followed, including pharmacological echo-stress, which resulted negative for ischemic cardiopathy, reason for which, the referring cardiologist advised against coronary angiography in favour of beta-blockers therapy. Family history and remote physiology resulted *unremarkable.* Resting electrocardiogram did not indicate pathological aspects. He thus underwent exercise stress testing on the cyclo-ergometer with increasing protocol. The exam unequivocally indicated anomalies of VR (ST segment depression in the horizontal type on anterolateral leads), typical for ischemia, brought on by medium-high external stress work load, associated with PVC and PSVC with secondary anomalies more highly accentuated in the VR. Subsequently the athlete was encouraged to undergo a coronary angiography, which later indicated the presence of critical calcified stenosis of the anterior interventricular branch of the left coronary artery, including the origin of two important diagonal branches , it furthermore indicated critical stenosis of the circumflex and critical stenosis of the second marginal narrow branch; dominant right coronary resulted clear. Consequently a silent bi-vessel coronopathy was diagnosed.

Therefore, the patient underwent percutaneous transluminal coronary angioplasty (PTCA) with medication on anterior intra ventricular branch of the left coronary artery on the middle segment and following PTCA with Kissing balloon technique on the second marginal branch. During that procedure, physicians indicated further PTCA procedure on circumflex coronary artery (CX).

Furthermore, the patient carried out another haemodynamic exam which indicated a progression of the coronary pathology with 50% stenosis of the common trunk, severe stenosis intrastent (/based on) IVA, D1 and D2; severe ostial of MO1.

The patient underwent myocardial revascularization via BRAC (direct with left internal mammary on anterior down sloping and sequential right mammary). The patient is today in great health and goes on cycling holidays.

Case 5 BSF (49 year-old male cyclist) non atherosclerotic coronaropathy (anomaly: double myocardial bridging on anterior descending artery)

Competitive cyclist who had undergone and passed fitness tests since 2002, despite the presence of certain aspects, at first aspecific and then dubious regarding right ventricular in the electrocardiogragraphic tracings, especially in 2005. Family history was positive for ischemic cardiopathy on his father's side.

Physiological case history: ex smoker, veteran competitive athlete (Km > 10,000 annually)

Pathological Anamnesis: left nephrectomy in 1979; fracture of left foot metatarsal and left elbow radius, clinically asymptomatic for 'chest pain', dyspnoea, asthenia, performance drop, etc... The patient underwent ECG at rest which indicated normal sinus rhythm with heart rate at 60 bpm, a vertical electric axis and aspecific anomalies of the on inferior lateral leads.

The exercise stress testing on the cycle-ergometer was carried out by maximum protocol of the increasing type adapted to mature competitive cyclists – warm up at 90 watts for 5 to 6 min with 30 watts increases at high revolutions up to an maximal external load of 270 watts – was interrupted at 8th minute on the appearance of the anomalies in the Ventricular Repolarization, in the lateral anterior region, fromV4 to V6 (ST depression from point J of 2-3 mm in a stress effort, with slow recovery of normal repolarization in the active recovery period at 75 watts. Physiological increase and decrease of arterial blood pressure.

The conclusion was therefore: evident signs of ischemic anomalies of the ventricular repolarization, at a high work load level (ECG findings decidedly worse than previous years) and in phase of non aerobic captation, cause for, according to guidelines, immediate coronary investigation not finalized solely to award the athlete his fitness certificate rather, in order to obtain a wider prognostic significance due to the suspected silent ischemic cardiopathy from probable obstructive coronaropathy (atherosclerotic or non atherosclerotic). Subsequently, the athlete had a coronary angiography which indicated a double muscular bridge of myocardial fibres on a down-sloping anterior, with classical imaging of coronary monitoring in the systolic stage.

Conclusion: The athlete was held unfit for competitive physical activity.

Case 6 B.B.(59 year old competitive amateur cyclist) Non critical mono-vessel proximal atherosclerotic coronary artery disease on descending artery (DA).

The athlete is an amateur cyclist who has always had in recent years , anomalies of the ventricular repolarization in the lateral anterior region, from V4 to V6 due to a ST segment depression of 1mm at 0.008seconds from point J, with slow ascending type pattern, causing doubts for ischemia brought on by stress efforts. The patient has always been asymptomatic. Family case history is positive for precocious ischemic cardiopathy (father died from myocardial infarction). On the other hand, no cardiovascular risk factors emerged. The athlete underwent the usual sport medicine protocol fitness test, in this case, for cycling. No anomalies were indicated in resting ECG*: sinus rhythm* at 80 bpm; intermediate electrical axis with aspecific anomalies of VR in anterior lateral leads. The test on the cyclometer at maximum effort was interrupted due to muscular exhaustion and for reaching a value of FC superior to FC theoretical max (> 110%).

From 6th minute of test anomalies began appearing of VR in the antero-lateral leads, (D1-AVLV5-V6) which reached a maximum level of the ST segment depression of about 3 mm at 0.05 ms from point J with firstly, a horizontal pattern, then a down-sloping one, between 9th and

10th minutes, corresponding to a maximum external work load (175 watts) with slow recovery of normal repolarization in the period of active recovery at 75 watt.

The patient was absolutely asymptomatic throughout the duration of the maximal test.

A notable worsening was seen in electrocardiographic anomalies compared to the tracings, carried out with same protocol, as in the previous years.

Such anomalies of the VR strongly indicative of myocardial ischemia, due to maximal effort at medium to high work load, reason for which, secondary level cardiological investigation was decided upon in order to exclude any suspicion of silent ischemic cardiopathy, therefore either myocardial scintigraphy or CT coronary multiple-slices.

One month later, the patient underwent angio -CT coronary 16 multiple-slices which indicated at IVA level, a calcified plaque of the proximal segment which determined non-significant stenosis (50%), that precociously forks into a diagonal branch lesion-free diagonal branch.

A similar, calcified plaque, not haemodynamically significant was found at crux.

Considering the existing recommendations concerning participation in competitive sports for athletes with cardiovascular disease, we advised carrying out a coronary angiography which the patient continued to disdain even on the advice of a trusted cardiologist .

Conclusions: as a precaution, seeing the unequivocal electrocardiographic proof of ischemia, brought on by effort and widespread endocardial damage, confirmed by the presence of atherosclerosis of the IVA proximal tract, it was decided not to give the athlete approval of fitness.

*Case 7(M.V.) Amateur Athlete Fidal (*Italian Federation of Athletics*), 60 yr old marathon runner.*
The athlete had been under control for a few years, concerning fitness assessment for running and marathon. Family history was positive for ischemic cardiopathy (his father had died at 56 from IMA; followed by two brothers who had died at 54 and 59 respectively).

The patient had arterial hypertension from light to moderate as well as hypercholesterolomy.

Prior examinations had always obtained negative results. Remote Anamnesis: Blind in Rx eye, due to an accident in childhood. The athlete had always been asymptomatic.

The athlete underwent a resting ECG which resulted within the normal limits and immediately after a maximal exercise testing on the treadmill following Bruce protocol.

The maximum test was interrupted at the 3rd step at a heart rate of 145 bpm, due to the appearance of polymorphous BEV and of the ST segment depression of 2mm at 0,08 sec from point J in the lower-lateral deviations, with signs of T-negative of inferior derivations during recovery time. This evidence of reduced coronary reserve caused us to move on to secondary level cardiological examinations, thus a pharmacological stress echocardiography was decided upon.

The athlete carried out the examination at a cardiac secondary level centre, using Dobutamine, which resulted negative for signs of inducible ischemia.

During a sport event the athlete who at the time was walking uphill complained of chest pain and dyspnea. The athlete, thus underwent a coronary angiography on 08.03.05, which indicated a serious multi-vessel coronary disease which required immediate re-vascularization with PTCA with placement of drug medical stent on the ostial circumflex (CX) artery branch; PTCA + 2 stent on second obtuse marginal branch; PTCA + 2 stent on first obtuse marginal branch.

He was also advised to undergo brief coronary revascularization via PTCA of the middle section of the Rx coronary, too. Two years later, the athlete is healthy and physically active .

FALSE POSITIVES

Case 8 (B.E.) 51year old amateur marathon runner (2006)

Family case history: father died at 75 from pancreatic cancer; 75 year old mother living, who suffers from hypertensive cardiopathy, aortic valvulopathy (stenosis) of a light to moderate entity, and more recently idiopathic pulmonary thromboembolism as well as macro-adenoma hypophisis, under pharmacological therapy.

Physiological anamnesis: adolescent smoker, drinks wine at meal times, and occasionally spirits; Triathlon athlete competitive from 30 to 40 years old and competitive long distance runner until a few years ago (last marathon run in 2003, Venice). Regularly trains, at least 3 times a week.

Recent remote pathological Anamnesis: Admitted at the age of 36, to Cesena Hospital, Internal Medicine Dept for DVS, in the left underarm area, following exams did not exclude the possibility of congenital Thrombophlebitis. A recent drop in athletic performance, respiratory breathlessness at the onset of physical exercise that resolves itself in 15 – 20 minutes. The objective exam was normal as were urine and spirography. The ECG at rest indicated normal sinus rhythm to Fc of 76 bpm normal intra-ventricular and atrioventricular conduction, mean electrical axis of QRS on the frontal surface of 45°, ventricular fibrillation trace, normal.

The following exercise stress testing on the cyclo-ergometer carried out for the first time with a triangular protocol adapted to competitive master athletes (ie, warm up at 50 – 70 watts for around 5, 6 minutes with 25 watt increases every 2° minute at high revolutions per minute up to a maximum external work load of 175 watts) was interrupted at the 12th minute on the appearance of abnormalities in the ventricular repolarization in the front lateral region, from V4 to V6 (ST segment depression at 0.08 sec from point J of 2 – 3 min with horizontal pattern – slow upward moving) suggestive of subendocardial ischemia, with slow recovery of normal repolarization in the phase of active recovery at 90 watts (see fig. 5)

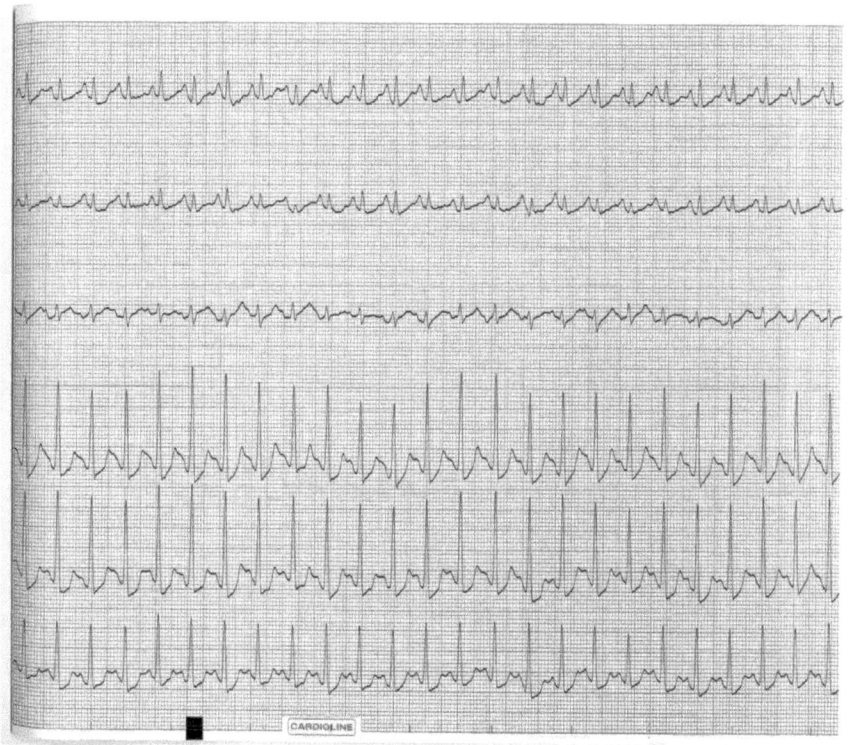

Figure 5

A further maximal exercise testing with a rectangular protocol was interrupted at 2° minute on the
appearance of the same, no slightly worse, abnormalities of the ventricular repolarization, in the
anterolateral (ST segment depression at 0.08 sec from point J in front lateral region (leads V4 – V6)
of about 3mm with a down-sloping pattern. In conclusion due to evidence of abnormalities of the
ventricular repolarization, of the ischemic type at work load of150-175 watt, in a person with case
history and clinical data including thrombophlebitis risk, require immediate coronary angiography
investigation, in order to exclude the presence of a critical monovasal obstructive coronaropathy,
The coronary angiography shows patent coronary artery. Well maintained overall contractibility of

the left ventricle. Permission to practice athletic and marathon running was given on the evidence of these facts.

Case 9 (F.F.) 66 year old amateur track athlete (2004)

Amateur athlete who had taken part in competitive track events for 20 years.

His case history included a moderate hypercholesterolemia, never adequately treated (no medicine, no specific diet for a sweet tooth), a Body Mass Index (BMI) over 27, and recently a central (abdominal) obesity, suggesting an insulin resistance. Furthermore chronic obstructive pulmonary disease (COPD), presently at stage 1 with a 15% ventilator deficit (mixed type), offset by chronic therapy including beta 2 stimulants and immune-stimulating therapy. The athlete after consent and warm up, underwent a stress test in ideal environmental conditions on the treadmill with continuous ECG monitoring, in 6 derivations, Bruce protocol. The test was interrupted shortly before the 10th minute (4th step) having reached theoretical maximal heart rate and on the appearance of abnormalities in the ST segment in the lateral leads (ST segment depression of the slow upward moving kind in V5 and square or horizontal kind in V6 around 2.6mm), with metabolic intensity running at 9,7 METS. The ST segment depression in the deviations mentioned resolved in the course of 3-6 minutes of recovery, firstly active, then passive. The arterial blood pressure values remained normal within accepted limits. The athlete was asymptomatic and not totally exhausted muscularly. This objective data, added to the clinical data regarding cardiovascular risk, obliged us to do further on the spot investigation, in particular cardiac catheterism with coronography in order to exclude mono-vessel coronary artery disease. Coronary angiography = Coronaries free from haemodynamically significant stenosis lesions. Permission to practice competitive activity and sport walking was granted.

Case 10 (M.M.) 55 years old highly competitive professional cyclist (2006)

The athlete came to the centre in order to renew fitness certificate for cycling. The athlete had been examined in the two previous years and had always passed. Family case history appeared insignificant and physiological anamnesis indicated intense sporting activity, high number of km covered (2000 km/year), a smoker in the past, type A personality structure. Recent and remote pathological anamnesis: appendicitis, a recent fracture of the left collar bone with consequent physical deconditioning (stop exercise from 30 – 40 days), sudden drops in athletic performance during competition. The Objective exam resulted normal; the resting ECG showed sinus bradycardia Heart Rate 56 bpm, left axial deviation, abnormalities of the ventricular repolarization. ABP = 125/80; Peripheral pulse in synchrony and normosphygmic. The exercise stress testing on the cycloergometer with maximal exercise protocol for competitive cyclists (i.e.setting off at 90 watts, with 30 watt increases a minute until stop and active recovery) was interrupted at 10th minute on appearance of significant electrocardiographic elements (ST depression at 0,08, from point J of 2 – 3 mm with down-sloping aspect)suggestive for ischemia brought on by maximum stress effort (heart rate 151 bpm, 90% theoretical maximal HR) with emphasis in the immediate recovery and slow reprise of a normal electrocardiographic aspect at the 6th minute at low external work load. Frequent premature ventricular contractions (PVCs), fusion beats, in pairs too, in warm-up stage as well as warm down. During the maximum test, the patient complained of presumed 'chest discomfort', what he described as dyspepsia (heart-burn). Further investigation was requested in the form of cardiac imaging, through myocardial scintigraphy with perfusion for maximum stress effort on cycloergometer in order to compare and make further ad hoc assessment. The perfusion did not indicate reversible deficit in capitation under maximum work load, however the unequivocal information, that settled the issue was the existence of a 48% ejection fraction (EF) after effort < 50% EF at rest. Such data indicated a light systolic deficit of the left ventricular, caused by suspect hyper-fusion (ischemia brought on by stress effort). In conclusion suspected pauci-symptomatic ischemic heart disease to be excluded or confirmed through ad hoc angiography (coronarography report = Coronaries free from significant haemodynamic stenosis lesions). The athlete was thus held to be fit for competitive sport activity.

Discussion

The predictive value of a system or diagnostic exam is not only correlated to sensitivity and specificity but also and above all to the probability a priori of signs of the disease in the people under investigation (probability pre-test) [27].

In an asymptomatic population it is logical to use an estimate of coronary heart disease risk through global assessment of cardiovascular risk according to the Framingham102 score, that places subjects in low, intermediate and high categories, taken from the third edition of ATP-III [3].

In order to improve the assessment of asymptomatic subjects at cardiovascular risk intermediate level, it is known that such individuals can benefit from further non-invasive tests like, for example the maximal stress test with ergometer, in order to obtain further information prognostically speaking, which will permit streamlining risk stratification [47].

Furthermore, in doubting a symptom or the positivity of a diagnostic test that might respect a false positive, carrying out a second test has greater predictive value, whether the result be positive or negative, in as much as the re-examined patient belongs to a selected group, whose probability pre-test is thus increased. As is common knowledge through the ECG exercise stress testing has a 78% sensitivity and 70% specifity, as a diagnostic method of coronary heart disease and 68% and 77% respectively for the European Society of Cardiology Test Force [22-82]. However, the maximal stress effort on specific ergometer is the most useful single test for recognizing silent myocardial ischemia, above all the context and setting of sports medicine, in consideration of the fact that for the members of the public examined (presumably it is a compulsory medical check-up for the healthy and asymptomatic). It is a cheap, standardized test, easily accessible and relatively safe (although requiring in the author's opinion, clearly defined protocols, suitable for maximum coronary reserve in Master athletes, who practice endurance sports [43 44 54].

Despite the fact that the application of the test is controversial and not accepted unanimously in assessing the screening of the asymptomatic general public due to the high number of false positives [43]. The ECG exercise stress testing remains the only method and possibility of action for sports medicine specialists, who are engaged in assessing physical exercise tolerance and cardiovascular functionality, or for any doctor cultivating an interest in preventive medicine.

So as to discover, for a wider prognostic significance too, elements affected by silent ischemic cardiopathy in marked advance in respect to the clinical manifestations of ischemic cardiopathy (angina, myocardial infarction, sudden death) [18-21-29].

This assumption is reported in the most recent American Guidelines on exercise stress testing, which places in class 2a asymptomatic diabetic patients who undertake vigorous physical exercise, and in class 2b the assessment of individuals suffering from multiple risk factors, males aged 45 and over, as well as females aged over 55, who carry out vigorous physical activity like for example Master athletes [45].

The exercise stress test interpretation depends both on analytical variability as well as the ability and experience of the operator, who has to be able to recognize and assess the eventual abnormalities in the ECG tracing (prevalently the pattern of the ST segment depression).

As proof of this, the different electrocardiographic signs registered in the same athletes by different physicians, in the various maximum tests they underwent in the 1st level check-up (maximal exercise stress testing on specific ergometer) and in the assessment of the 2nd level cardiological stress effort myocardial scintigraphy on the cycle ergometer).

In fact, in the course of the maximal exercise stress tests carried out under ad hoc protocol in the sports medicine centre, significant abnormalities in the ST segment emerge in clinical cases 2 and 3 (real positive tests), whilst in the course of the maximum ergometric test relative to the stress effort scintigraphy carried out in the 2nd level cardiological centre following a different protocol (classic cardiologic with increasing 25 watt steps every minute), no significant abnormalities in the ST segment were revealed (false negative tests), even with the evidence of perfusion deficit obtained in the immediately following scintigraphic exam.

It follows that the electrocardiographic tracing made by the cardiologist who carried out the stress effort scintigraphy, makes no real impact on any clinical decision, on the other hand the signs of evident defects in the myocardial perfusion represent important data in as much as they are correlated to myocardial ischemia. Solely in the case of the first athlete, who suffered from a serious critical disease of the common trunk, was there a clear electrographic concordance among the maximum tests, carried out in both 1st and 2nd level centres.

In cases 4 and 7, the athletes' 2nd level cardiological exams (pharmacological echocardiographic stress) were negative, but that fact did not mislead the clinical procedure and the prescription for the coronary angiography, as it hadn't been considered reliable enough.

In cases 5 and 6, it was decided to proceed directly to coronary angiography or a computerized tomography (CT) coronary angiogram, after the first level examination, with the intent of obtaining certainties or confirming personal considerations, both clinical and electrocardiographic, as well as speeding up diagnostic procedures, which are notably complicated in cases of presumed silent ischemic cardiopathy, being convinced that even in case of negative cardiological imaging (CT), that factor would not have dispelled any doubts, guaranteeing the certainty necessary for competitive fitness certification.

Silent ischemic cardiopathy is in fact, a complicated diagnosis, not an easy one, extremely delicate because the excessive possibility of erroneously casting a healthy athlete, as a sick person. That said, a MRFIT [76] [95] test has clearly demonstrated that asymptomatic males who obtained positive results from a stress effort test, have a cardiovascular risk event (angina pectoris, myocardial infarction, sudden death) 15 times superior (5 times, for women) to subjects who obtain negative results.

Nevertheless, the Seattle Heart Watch Study [13], reported asymptomatic males > 40 with one

coronary risk factor and at least 2 abnormalities, observed in the stress effort ECG, run an increased

risk of having cardiovascular events in a 5 year period, of 30 times superior compared to normal

individuals. It follows therefore that 1st level sport medicine specialists on becoming aware of, in

the reading of ECG during maximum effort test, abnormalities of ventricular repolarization,

extremely suggestive of myocardial ischemia brought on by stress effort, in Master athletes who

present cardiovascular risk factors which greatly increase the probability of coronary atherosclerotic

disease, are obliged not to underestimate such evidence and procedures, scientifically and morally

speaking, through further investigation in terms of imaging (myocardial scintigraphy, and should it

be necessary echo-stress) in order to discover the presence of silent ischemic cardiopathy, so as to

obtain more extensive prognostic meaning. The eventual benefits pertaining to myocardial

revascularization surgery in individuals suffering from stable atherosclerotic coronary heart disease

has been a part of animated discussion for many years, due to a wide number of controversial

studies, therefore it has not been simple to define optimum procedure strategy in a surgical or

preventive sense. The aim of this thesis has not only been to define strategies and above all

diagnostic procedures that sport medicine specialists, experts in sport cardiology, should undertake,

as well as pointing out the usefulness of accompanying these individuals, highly competitive

athletes, who suddenly find themselves as patients in follow-up procedures. The procedure of the

clinical cases discussed in this thesis for example, confirms the clinical formulation based on the

advantages of myocardial revascularization in highly selected patients and identified as regards to

medical therapy as also reported by Davies and alt in their ACIP [24] study, in which it is

demonstrated how aggressive treatment improves the prognosis of these patients, as is reported in

Thomas Killip's editorial on Circulation [60].These assumptions have been confirmed by Herrmann

HC [52] who points out how these are the first data that indicate an advantage in survival after

myocardial revascularization.

The same 1993 guidelines of ACC/AHA reviewed in 2001[1], recommend PTCA surgery. In class 1, in those asymptomatic diabetic individuals with more than one significant coronary lesion in one or two blood vessels, In class IIb, in asymptomatic individuals, with significant lesions in at least 3 arteries open to revascularization and a high success probability with low surgical risk. In class III in asymptomatic subjects who did not fit into the criteria of classes I and II and who have got, amongst the various options, critical stenosis of left ventricular descending artery. In fact, the patients involved in case histories 1 – 3 – 4 – 7 (true positives) underwent myocardial revascularization surgery via BPAC in the critical lesion of the common trunk (case 1); in first instance with PTCA then with BPAC in the patient with critical multi-vessel disease (case 4); with PTCA + stent for multi-vessel disease (case 7); and with PTCA + stent for proximal bi-vessel disease of the DA and 1st ostial branch (case 3). As for the patient in case 2, the consulting cardiologist decided on conservative pharmacological therapy as the bi-vessel coronary disease was not of a critical condition, whilst in case 5, the tracings of the patient (double myocardial bridge) have been lost due to interfering colleagues and in case 6, it was decided the patient should undertake a course of conservative therapy for presumed non-critical mono-vessel disease, not properly investigated with coronary angiography. The results of MASS II [99] Study have recently been published which indicate a significant reduction of the primary end point (death) in 5 years of follow up in patients who surgically underwent BPAC for multi-vessel disease.

Even if the possible benefits of myocardial revascularization surgery, in the treatment of asymptomatic individuals, such as athletes, with stable atherosclerotic coronary artery disease, will always be disputed and not always decided upon immediately, it appears obvious to hold that for greater myocardial revascularization following BPCA or PTCA procedures heralds a better prognosis compared to conservative pharmacological therapy, and thus the physician can safely permit resumption of sporting activity on the part of the athlete [24 56 72].

Conclusions

The relationship, both positive and negative, between cardiac ischemic disease (CHD) and physical activity remains a central issue. Incidence and severity of CHD increase linearly with aging, reaching maximal levels around age 50 years in men and in postmenopausal women.

Coronary atherosclerosis is the most common form of heart disease relevant to the Master population as a cause of sudden cardiac death, with a reported prevalence of up to 90-100% [65-67].

In addition, although several studies have consistently demonstrated that regular physical activity protects patients from coronary events, strenuous exertion may trigger myocardial infarction as a result of acute thrombotic occlusion, following intimal bleeding and/or plaque rupture in coronary arteries that were not previously critically narrowed. The relative risk of myocardial infarction increases exponentially in sedentary individuals not accustomed to high-intensity exercise.

In conclusion, the diagnostic procedure of an athlete, who, even in the absence of any symptomatology, presents abnormalities in ventricular repolarization, during a maximal exercise stress testing in 1st level examination thus suggesting stress effort myocardial ischemia. It is a difficult procedure, obstacle ridden, urging however further investigation and which should thus be treated with the same commitment and obligations as those individuals with similar ischemia brought on by stress effort, however symptomatic [74].

In any case, as COCIS 2003 [20], states, the non-disappearance or ex-novo appearance of ARV (ventricular repolarization abnormalities) demand further investigation, to ascertain or exclude the presence of ischemic cardiopathy, above all in sportsmen > 35 – 40 years old and/or with increased cardiovascular risk.

In short, the author, on the basis of personal experience, takes the liberty of observing, the following:

- Maximal exercise ECG stress testing is the main examination, in screening Master athletes as Zeppilli [103] states;

- The diverse electrocardiographic response from the maximal ergometric stress tests in the cases described, always positive in the protocol utilized by the sports specialists and often negative in the maximum tests carried out by the nuclear-imaging cardiologist also in the presence of perfusional deficits, make some people hold that the protocol to be used should absolutely be of the incremental triangular type, and foresee increasing loads of short duration, which do not permit the accumulation of peripheral fatigue and reaching maximum consumption of oxygen in a short period of time after adequate warm-up and therefore surmount the anaerobic threshold (which, in highly competitive Master athletes is close to maximum consumption of oxygen and therefore often well over 85/90% maximum theoretical heart rate [23 89]), but also that examination procedure has to be personalized and adapted to the anthrop-morphological and physiological characteristics of the athlete;

- the second cardiac imaging test to use is preferably the myocardial scintigraphy, or rather a perfusion test, appropriately carried out by the maximum-stress effort protocol [83];

- it is held in fact, pharmacological echo-stress is a method dependent on the operator's skill (and is also chest dependent) and despite literature indicates a greater specificity respect to the scintigraphy this regards the comparison of the two methods by means of the use of the stress effort test, and non-pharmacological, it is clear that diagnostic reliability (ergo its predictive ability) depends on who is doing the exam;

- In case of evidence, even a light perfusional deficit indicated in the myocardial scintigraphy, it is absolutely necessary to study in depth, with an invasive coronary investigation, above all in the presence of other eventual cardiovascular risk factors; the procedure with negative scintigraphy urges further research.

Recently, multislice computed tomography (CT) has been shown to be capable of visualizing not only the coronary arteries (wall and lumen), but also the cardiac muscle, with high spatial resolution [79]. Multislice CT provides high-quality three-dimensional images of

48

coronary arteries. Initial results of four-, 16- and more recently 64-slice CT, compared with conventional angiograms, are very promising. Non invasive visualization of the coronary arteries and accurate detection of stenosis are now possible with ECG-gated 16-slice CT [103]. Multislice CT can also detect nonstenotic coronary plaques. Electron beam tomography coronary calcium imaging is an evolving technique for the early detection of coronary atherosclerosis, and recent studies have established its prognostic value in asymptomatic individuals. The relationship of coronary artery calcium scores to obstructive CAD is an evolving area of interest and is clinically relevant because it determines which individuals are likely to benefit from revascularization procedures.

The coronary angiography remains the golden standard in the diagnosis of silent ischemic cardiopathy [98], even if the evidence of coronaries free from the obstructive atherosclerotic process does not eliminate the doubt of an ischemic genesis of the electrocardiographic aspects of subendocardial ischemia, as it does not explain the cause of the ST segment depression, however it does guarantee fitness approval for sport [99].

The personal record of cases of the authors confirms the importance of cardiological screening for sportsmen and women, above all in Master Athletes, as it is well known that ischemic heart disease is the principal cause of cardiac pathology at risk of sudden death in Master Athletes (over 35, in age) and predominantly strikes the male sex, as stated by Corrado and co-authors [22].

Silent myocardial ischemia is a major challenge for physicians, especially for sports doctors and sports cardiologists, because the disease is known to everyone although recognizing it, is a true state of the art.

Bibliography

1. *ACC/AHA Guidelines for Percutaneous Coronary Intervention (Revision of the 1993 PTCA Guidelines) A report of the American College of Cardiology/American Heart Association Task Force on Practice Guidelines. IACC Vol.37. No. 8, 2001 June 15,2001*

2. *ACC/AHA Guideline Update for Exercise Testing. Summary Article: A Report of the American College of Cardiology/American Heart Association Task Force on Practice Guidelines (Committee to Update the 1997 Exercise Testing Guidelines) Circulation. 2002; 106: 1883 – 1892*

3. *Adult Treatment Panel III. Expert panel on Detection, Evaluation, and Treatment of High Blood Cholesterol in Adults. Executive summary of the third report of the National Cholesterol Education Program (NCEP). Jama. 2001;285:2486-2497*

4. *Allen, W.K., Seals, D.R., Hurley, B.F., Ehsani, A.A. and Hagberg, J.M. (1985) Lactate threshold and distance running performance in young and older endurance athletes. Journal of Applied Physiology 58, 1281-1284.*

5. *American Academy of Family Physicians. Age charts for periodic health examination. Kansas City, MO: American Academy of Family Physicians, 1994.*

6. *American College of Cardiology/American Heart Association. Guidelines for electrocardiography. A report of the American College of Cardiology/American Heart Association Task Force on Assessment of Diagnostic and Therapeutic Cardiovascular Procedures (Committee on Electrocardiography). J Am Coll Cardiol 1992;19:473-481*

7. *American College of Sports Medicine. Guidelines for exercise testing and prescription. 4th ed. Philadelphia: Lea & Febiger, 1991*

8. *Balady G, Larson M, Vasan R, Leip EP, O'Donnel C, Levy D.Usefulness of exercise testing in the prediction of coronary disease risk among asymptomatic person as a function of the Framingham risk score.; Circulation 2004 Oct 5; 110(14): 1920-5. Epub 2004 Sep 27. (abstract)*

9. *Basilico FC. Cardiovascular disease in athetes. Am J Sports Med 1999;27:108-21*

10. *Beckerman J, Mathur A, Stahr S, Myers J, Chun S, Froelicher V. Exercise-induced ventricular arrhythmias and cardiovascular death. Ann Noninvasice Electrocardiol. 2005 Jan;10(1):47-52*

11. *Begum S, Katzel LI. Silent ischemia during voluntary detraining and future cardiac events in master athletes. Am Geriatr Soc 2000 Jun;48:647-50*

12. *Biagini E, Schinkel AF, Bax JJ, et al. Long term outcome in patients with silent versus symptomatic ischaemia during dobutamine stress echocardiography. Heart 2005;91:737-42*

13. *Bruce RA, Hossack KF, DeRouen TA, Hofer V. Enhanced risk assessment for primary coronary heart disease events by maximal testing ; 10 years' experience of Seattle Heart Watch. J Am Coll Cardiol. 1983;2:565-73*

14. *Bruce RA, DeRouen TA, Hossack KF. Value of maximal exercise test in risk assessment of primary coronary disease events in healthy men. Five years' experience of the Seattle heart watch study. Am J Cardiol. 1980; 46: 371-378*

15. *Callaham P, Froelicher VF, Klein J, Risch M, Dubach P, Friis R. Exercise-induced silent ischaemia: Age, diabetes mellitus, previous myocardial infarction and prognosis. J Am Coll Cardiol 1989;14:1175-1180*

16. *Canadian Task Force on the Periodic Health Examination. The periodic health examination: 1984 update. Can Med Assoc J 1984;130:2-15*

17. *Cohn PF. Silent myocardial ischemia. Ann Intern Med 1988;109:312-317.*

18. *Cohn PF, Fox K, Daly C. Silent Myocardial Ischemia. Circulation 2003; 108:1263-1277*

19. *Cohn PF, Gorlin R, Vokonas PS, Williams RA, Herman MV. A quantitative clinical index for the diagnosis of symptomatic coronary artery disease. N Engl J Med 1972;286:901-907*

20. *Comitato Organizzativo Cardiologico Per L'Idoneità Allo Sport (COCIS). Protocolli cardiologici per il giudizio dell'idoneità sportiva agonistica 2003. Casa Editrice Scientifica Internazionale Roma*

21. *Conti CR. Silent cardiac ischemia. Current Opinion in Cardiology 2002; 17:537-542*

22. *Corrado D, Pelliccia A, Bjornstad HH, ThieneG. Cardiovascular pre-participation screening of young competitive athletes for prevention of sudden death: proposal for a common European protocol. Eur Heart J 2005; 26:516-524*

23. *Costill DL, Fink WJ, and Pollok ML. Muscle fibre composition and enzyme activities of elite distance runner. Medicine Science Sport and Exercise. 1976;8:96-100*

24. *Davies RF, Goldberg AD, Forman S, Pepine CJ, Knatterud GL, Geller N, Sopko G, Pratt C, Deanfield J, Conti CR, for the ACIP Investigators. Asymptomatic Cardiac Ischemia Pilot (ACIP) Study two-year follow-up: outcomes of patients randomized to initial strategies of medical therapy versus revascularization. Circulation. 1997;95:2037-2043*

25. *Detrano R, Gianrossi R, Froelicher V. The diagnostic accuracy of the exercise electrocardiogram: a meta-analysis of 22 years of research, Prog. Cardiovasc Dis 1989; 32:173-206)*

26. *Detrano R, Froelicher V. A logical approach to screening for coronary artery disease. Ann Intern Med 1987;106:846-852*

27. *Detrano R, Yiannikas J, Salcedo EE, et al.: Bayesan probability analysis: A prospective demonstration of its clinical utility in diagnosis coronary disease. Circulation 1984; 69:541*

28. *Diamond GA. How accurate is SPECT thallium scintigraphy? J Am Coll Cardiol 1990;16:1017-1021*

29. *Droste C, Ruf G, Greenlee MW, et al.: Development of angina pectoris pain and cardiac events in asymptomatic patients with myocardial ischemia. Am J Cardiol. 1993, 72:121-127*

30. *Eddy DM, ed. Common screening tests. Philadelphia: American College of Physicians, 1991:398-401*

31. *Ekelund LG, Suchindran C, McMahon RP, et al. Coronary Heart disease morbidity and mortality in hypercholesterolemic men predicted from an exercise test: The Lipid Research Clinics Coronary Primary Prevention Trial. J Am Coll Cardiol. 1989; 14:556-563*

32. *Epstein S. Quyyumi A, Bonow R. Myocardial ischemia: silent or symptomatic. N Eng J Med. 1988; 318:1038-1043*

33. *Epstein SE, Quyumi A, Bonow RO. Sudden cardiac death without warning: possible mechanisms and implications for screening asymptomatic populations. N Engl J Med 1989;321:320-323.*

34. *Erikssen J, Enge I, Forfang J, Shorstein O. False-positive diagnostic tests and coronary angiographic findings in 105 presumably healthy males. Circulation. 1976;54:371-376*

35. *Erikksen J, Thaulow E. Follow up of patients with asymptomatic myocardial ischaemia. In: Rutishauser W, Roskamm H, eds. Silent Myocardial Ischaemia. Berlin, Germany: Springer-Verlag, 1984:154-164*

36. *European Guidelines on Cardiovascular Disease Prevention in Clinical Practice. Third Joint Task Force of European and other Societies on Cardiovascular Disease Prevention in Clinical Practice. European Journal of Cardiovascular Prevention and Rehabilitation 2003, 10, (Suppl.1): S1-S78*

37. *Executive Summary of the Screening for Heart Attack Prevention and Education – SHAPE-Task Force Report. Am J Cardiol 2006; 98(suppl): 2H-15H*

38. *Fleg JL, Gerstenblith G, Zonderman AB, et al. Prevalence and prognostic significance of exercise-induced silent myocardial ischemia detected by thallium scintigraphy and electrocardiography in asymptomatic volunteers. Circulation 1990;81:428-436.*

39. *Fleg JL. Prevalence and prognostic significance of exercise-induced silent myocardial ischemia in apparently healthy subjects. Am J Cardiol 1992 Mar 6;69(7):14B-18*

40. *Fleisch M. Exercise echocardiography or exercise SPECT imaging ? A meta-analysis of diagnostic test performance. Jama 1998 Sep 9;280(10):913-20*

41. Fletcher,G.F.,M.D. and Schlant,R.C.,The Exercise Test, Hurst's The Heart,8th Edition,P.423-440.)

42. Fortuin NJ, Weiss JL. Exercise stress testing. Circulation 1977;56-699-721

43. Fowler-Brown A, Pignone M, Pletcher M, Tice JA, Sutton SF, Lohr KN; U.S. Preventive Task Force. Exercise tolerance testing to screen for coronary artery disease: a systematic review for the technical support for the U.S. Preventive Services Task Force. Ann Intern Med. 2004; 140: W9-W24

44. Gianrossi R, Detrano R, Mulvihill D, et al. Exercise-induced ST depression in the diagnosis of coronary artery disease: a meta-analysis. Circulation 1989;80:87-98

45. Gibbons RJ, et al. ACC/AHA 2002 Guidelines Update for Exercise Testing. A Report of the American College of Cardiology/American Heart Association Task Force on Practice Guidelines (Committe to Update the 1997 Exercise Testing Guidelines). Circulation 2002;106:1883-1892

46. Greenberg PS, Friscia DA, Ellestad MII. Predictive accuracy of Q-X/Q-T ratio, Q-Tc interval, S-T depression and R wave amplitude during stress testing. Am J Cardiol 1997; 44:18-23

47. Greenland P, Smith SG Jr, Grundy SM. Improving coronary heart disease risk assessment in asymptomatic people: role of traditional risk factors and noninvasive cardiovascular tests. Circulation. 2001; 104:1863-1867.)

48. Guidelines of the management of stable angina pectoris: executive summary. Task Force on the Management of Stable Angina Pectoris of European Society of Cardiology. European Heart Journal (2006) 27; 1341 -1 841

49. Harris CN, Aronow WS, Parker DP, et al. Treadmill stress test in left ventricular hypertrophy. Chest 1973; 63:353-357

50. Heller LI, Tresgallo M, Sciacca RR, et al.: Prognostic significance of silent myocardial ischemia on a thallium stress test. Am J Cardiol. 1990, 65:718-721

51. Hellerstein IIK, Prozan GB, Leibow IM, et al. The two-step exercise test as a test of cardiac function in chronic rheumatic heart disease and in arteriosclerotic heart disease with old myocardial infarction- Am J Cardiol 1961;7:234-252

52. Herrmann HC. Revascularization Best for Silent Ischemia. Journal Watch Cardiology, May 19, 1997; 1997 (579):1-1

53. Hood S, Northcote RJ. Cardiac assessment of veteran endurance athletes: a 12 years follow up study. Br J Sports Med 1999;33:239-243

54. Ilic D, Ilic MD, Petrovic D, Tasic I, Djordjevic D, Bojan I. Silent Myocardial Ischemia in Asymptomatic Patients With Multiple Coronary Risk Factors. Medicine and Biology. 2004; 11(3):107-112

55. *Josephson RA[1], Shefrin E, Lakatta EG, Brant LJ, Fleg JL.. Can serial exercise testing improve the prediction of coronary events in asymptomatic individuals ? Circulation. 1990;81:21-24 -*

56. *Katritsis DG, Ioannidis J. Percutaneous Coronary Intervention Versus Conservative Therapy in Nonacute Coronary Artery Disease_ A meta-Analysis. Circulation. 2005;111:2906-2912*

57. *Katzel LI, Fleg Jerome L, Busby-Whitehead J, Sorkin J, Becker LC, Lakatta EG, ans Golberg AP. Exercise-induced Silent Myocardial Ischemia in Master Athletes. Am J Cardiol 1998;81:261-265*

58. *Kaul P, Fu Y, Ching Chamg WC, Harrington R, Moliterno DJ, Van dw Werf F, Armstrong PW. The ST depression > o = 2mm sign: An ominous prognosis in acute coronary syndromes. Circulation 1999;100:1497-1504*

59. *Kemp HG, Kronmal RA, Vlietstra RE, Frye FL. Seven year survival of patients with normal or near normal coronary arteriograms: a CASS registry study. J Am Coll Cardiol 1986;7:479-483*

60. *KillipThomas. Silent Myocardial Ischemia: Some Good News. Circulation. 1997;95:1992-1993*

61. *Kligfield P, Lauer M. Exercise Electrocardiogram Testing. Beyond the ST Segment. Circulation 2006; 114:2070-2082*

62. *Kotler TS, Diamond GA. Exercise thallium-201 scintigraphy in the diagnosis and prognosis of coronary artery disease. Ann Intern Med 1990;113:684-702*

63. *Kujala UM, Sarna S, Kaprio J, et al. Heart attacks and lower-limb function in master endurance athletes. Med Sci Sports Exerc. 1999;31:1041-1046*

64. *Lauer MS. Exercise electrocardiogram testing and prognosis: novel markers and predictive instruments. Cardiol Clin. 2001;19:401-414*

65. *Laukkanen JA, Kurl S, Lakka T, er al. Exercise-induced silent myocardial ischemia and coronary morbidity and mortality in middle-aged men. J Am Coll Cardiol. 2001; 38:72-79*

66. *Lee IM, Hsieeh CC, Paffermbarger RS Jr. Exercise intensity and longevity in men: the Harvard Alumni Heath Study. Jama 1995;273: 1179-1184*

67. *Maron BJ, Epstein SE, Roberts WC. Causes of sudden death in competitive athletes. J Am Coll Cardiol 1986;7:204-14*

68. *Maron BJ, Araùjo CG, Thompson PD, Fletcher GF, Bayès de Luna A, Fleg J, Pelliccia A, Balady GJ, Furlanello F, Van Camp SP, Elosua R, Chaitman BR, Bazzarre TL. Recommendations for Preparticipation Screening and the Assessment of Cardiovascular Disease in Master Athletes – An advisory for Healtcare Professionals From the Working Groups of the World Heart Federation of Sports Medicine, and the American Heart*

Association Committee on Exercise, Cardiac Rehabilitation, and Prevention. Circulation 2001;103:327-334)

69. Mattingly TW. The post-exercise electrocardiogram: its value in the diagnosis and prognosis of coronary artery disease. Am J Cardiol 1962; 9:395-409

70. McHenry PL, Fisch C. Clinical applications of the treadmill exercise test. Mod Concepts Cardiovasc Dis 1977; 46:21-25

71. Mittelman MA, Maclure M, Tofler GH, at al. Triggering of acute myocardial infarction by heavy physical exertion: protection against triggering by regular exertion: Determinants of Myocardial Infarction Onset Study Investigators. N Eng J Med. 1993;329:1677-1683

72. Mitten MJ, Maron BJ. Legal considerations affecting medical eligibility for competitive athletes with cardiovascular abnormalities and acceptance of Bethesda Conference on Sports Eligibility Recommendations. J Am Coll Cardiol 1994; 24:861-3

73. Morton E. Travel. Stress Testing in Cardiac Evaluation: Current Concepts with Emphasis on the ECG. Chest 2001; 119:907-925

74. Mulcahy DA. The return of silent ischaemia ? Not really. Heart 2005;91:1249-1250

75. Murray CJ, Lopez AD. Alternative projections of mortality and disability by cause 1990-2020: Global Burden of Disease Study. Lancet. 1997; 349:1498-1504.

76. Neaton JD, Wentworth D. Serum cholesterol, blood pressure, cigarette smoking, and death from coronary heart disease. Overall findings and differences by age for 316,099 white men. Multiple Risk Factor Intervention Trial Research Group. Arch Intern Med 1992 Jan;152(1):56-64

77. Noakes TO, Opie LH, Rose AG, et al. Autopsy-proved coronary atherosclerosis in marathon runners. N Eng J Med 1979; 301:86-89

78. Parmley W.W. Prevalence and clinical significance of silent myocardial ischemia. Circulation 1989 Dec;80(6 Suppl):IV68-73

79. Pasternak RC, Abrams J, Greenland P, Smaha LA, Wilson PW. Houston Miller N. 34th Bethesda Conference: task force#1-Identification of coronary artery disease risk: is there a detection gap ? J Am Cardiol. 2003; 41:1863-1874

80. Pasternak RC, et al. Identification of coronary artery disease risk: is there a detection gap? J Am Cardiol. 2003; 41:1863-1874.

81. Pelliccia A, Maron BJ. Pre-participation cardiovascular evaluation of the competitive athlete: perspectives from the 30 years Italian experience. Am J Cardiol. 1995;75:827-829

82. Pelliccia A, Fagard R, Bjornstad HH, Anastassakis A, Arbustini E, Assanelli D, Biffi A, Borjesson M, Carrè F, Corrado D, Delise P, Dorwarth U, Hirt A, Heidbuchel H, Hoffmann E, Mellwig KP, Panhuyzen-Goedkoop N, Pisani A, Solberg EE, Van-Buuren F, and Vanhees

L. Recommendations for competitve sports participation in athletes with cardiovascular disease. A consensus document from the Study Group of Sports Cardiology of the Working group of Cardiac Rehabilitation and Exercise Physiology and the Working Group of Myocardial and Pericardial diseases of the European Society of Cardiology. European Heart Journal 2005;26:1422-1445

83. Pieri PL. Clinical decision making in patients with stable anginal symptoms: combining functional assessment with morphology to guide treatment. Eur J Nucl Med Mol Imaging 2005. 32:1360-1362

84. Pigozzi F, Spataro A, Alabiso A, Parisi A, Rizzo M, Fagnani F, Di Salvo V, Massazza G, Maffulli N. Role of exercise stress test in master athletes. Br J Sports Med 2005; 39:527-531

85. Okin PM, Kligfield P. Heart rate adjustment of ST segment depression and performance of the exercise electrocardiogram: a clinical evaluation. J Am Coll Cardiol. 1995;25:1726-1735

86. Ragosta M, Crabtree J, Sturner WQ, et al. Death during recreational exercise in the State of Rhode Island. Med Sci Sports Exerc. 1984;16:339-342

87. Rose G, Baxter PJ, Reid DD, McCartney P. Prevalence and prognosis of electrocardiographic findings in middle-aged men. Br Heart J 1978;40:636-643.

88. Rywik TM, Zink RC, Gittings NS, Kahn AA, Wright JG, O'connor FC, Fleg JL. Independent prognostic significance of ischeamic ST-segment responce limited recovery from treadmill exercise in asymptomatic subjects. Circulation 1998;97:2117-2122)

89. Saltin B, Nazer K, Costill DL, Stein E, Jansson E, Essen B, and Gollnick PD. The nature of the training response; peripheral and central adaptation to one legged exercise. Acta Physiologica Scandinavica. 1976; 96:289-305

90. Seto CK. Pre-participation cardiovascular screening. Clin Sports Med. 2003 Jan; 22(1):23-35

91. Siscovick DS, Weiss NS, Fletcher RH, et al. The incidence of primary cardiac arrest during vigorous exercise. N Eng J Med. 1984; 311:874-877)

92. Shlomo Stern. State of the Art in Stress Testing and Ischaemia Monitoring. Cardiac Electrophysiology Review 2002;6:204-208

93. Smith RII, LePetri B, Moisa RB, et al. Association of increased left ventricular mass in the absence of electrocardiographyc left ventricular hypertrophy with ST depression during exercise. Am J Cardiol 1995;76:973-974

94. Sox HC Jr, Garber AM, Littenberg B. The resting electrocardiogram as a screening test: a clinical analysis. Ann Intern Med 1989;111:489-502

95. Stamler J, Wentworth D, Neaton JD. Is relationship between serum cholesterol and risk of premature death from coronary heart disease continuous and graded? Findings in 356,222 primary screenees of the Multiple Risk Factor Intervention Trial (MRFIT). JAMA 1986 Nov 28;256(20):2823-8

96. *Stuart RJ, Ellestad MII. Upsloping ST segment in exercise testing. Am J Cardiol. 1976; 37:19-22*

97. *Schwartz RS, Jackson WG, Celio PV, Richardson LA, Hickman JR Jr. Accuracy of exercise 201-Tl myocardial scintigraphy in asymptomatic young men. Circulation 1993;87:165-172.*

98. *Thaulow E, Erikssen J, Sandvik L, Erikssen G, Jorgensen L, Cohn PF. Initial clinical presentation of cardiac disease in asymptomatic men with silent myocardial ischemia and angiographically documented coronary artery disease (the Oslo Ischemia Study). Am J Cardiol 1993;72:629-633.*

99. *Whady Hueb et al. Five-Year Follow –up of the Medicine, Angioplasty, or Surgery Study (MASS II) Circulation. 2007;115:1082-1089*

100. *Whang W, Manson JE, Hu FB et al. Physical exertion, exercise, and sudden cardiac death in women. Jama 2006;295:1399-1403*

101. *Willich SN, Lewis M, Lowel H, et al. Physical exertion as a trigger of acute myocardial infarction: Triggers and Mechanisms of Myocardial Infarction Study Group. N Eng J Med. 1993;329:1684-1690*

102. *Wilson PWF, D'Agostino RB, Levy D, et al. Prediction of coronary heart disease using risk factors categories. Circulation. 1998;97:1837-1847*

103. *Zeppilli Paolo. Cardiologia dello Sport. Terza Edizione 2001. Casa Editrice Scientifica Internazionale*

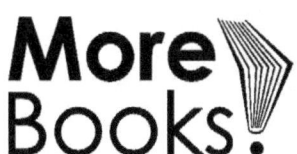
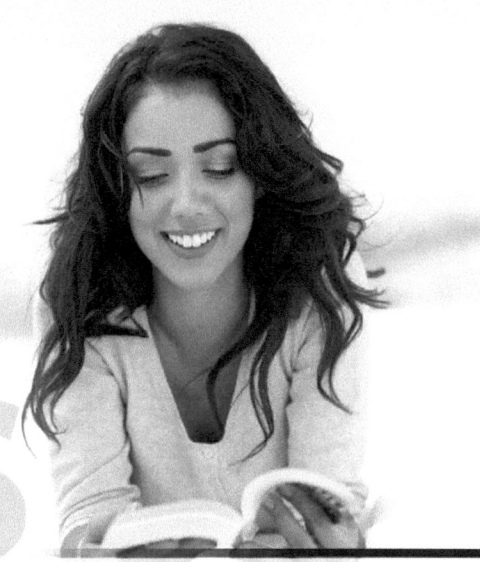
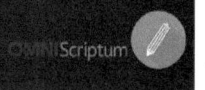

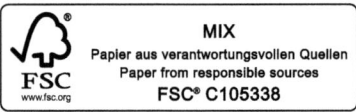
Printed by Books on Demand GmbH, Norderstedt / Germany